BETTER THAN HABITS

Greater Intelligence, Not Work

By

Robert S. Elliott

DISCLAIMER

Table of Contents

INTRODUCTION

Routines and systems can change people's lives.

Many individuals often mention habits as the cornerstone of success in personal development. However, the efficiency of routines and systems often outweighs the traditional emphasis on habits. Although habits are unquestionably crucial in shaping behavior, the application of routines and procedures can lead to significant personal change.

Because of their automaticity and subconscious nature, habits have garnered extensive investigation and support as the key to achieving goals. Repetitive behaviors that become ingrained in a person's daily routine form habits. The disadvantages of habits emerge from their concentration on behavior repetition rather than investigating the underlying mechanisms that underpin these behaviors. Routines and systems are a more complex method that goes beyond simply developing habits. Systems are more than simply frameworks; they are comprehensive strategies made up of a defined collection of interconnected behaviors that work together to achieve a certain purpose. Their core idea is to create an environment that encourages desirable actions rather than relying solely on repetition or willpower These systems make use of routines, which are a subset of systems. They bring order, structure, and rhythm to everyday life. Routines arrange a symphony of actions, compressing various behaviors and chores into a coherent sequence, whereas habits are typically based on single actions. The main difference is that routines and systems are proactive.

Systems go beyond habits and address the environment, triggers, and motivations that drive behaviors. They comprise a determined plan for creating an environment conducive to success in accomplishing the intended objectives. Take fitness and health as examples. It is beneficial to make going to the gym a regular habit. Still, a system should take a more comprehensive approach, including nutrition planning, workout scheduling, goal setting, and establishing a supportive environment. Routines are then used to make this strategy easier to implement, such as designating specific days and times for exercise, prepping meals ahead of time, and sticking to a predetermined schedule.

Furthermore, routines and systems are more adaptable than habits. In addition, people can adjust, alter, and tailor routines and systems to match changing needs and goals. This adaptability is critical in a changing world because it allows people to alter direction, enhance, and refine their plans without jeopardizing their objectives. In addition, routines and systems have a strong psychological impact. Automating chores, they lessen Decision fatigue and free up mental space for creativity and higher-order thinking. Systems allow workers to focus on strategic planning and innovation by reducing the cognitive load associated with frequent decision-making by embedding desired behaviors within a framework.

It is undeniable that routines, systems, and habits function together. Though habits are an essential aspect of everyday life, routines, and systems propel human development to new heights. They complement one another; routines and systems provide the infrastructure that supports and amplifies the influence of habits, which serve as the foundation. the current emphasis on habits in personal growth needs to include the power of routines and systems to change. Although habits are beneficial, including routines and systems in one's life, offers a diverse approach to achieving goals. People may create successful environments and break free from the confines of ingrained behavior by using the power of routines and systems to affect major long-term changes in their lives.

Chapter One

Life's Resources.

Life's Resources Are a Gold Mine Of Opportunities. Life's magnificent design creates a mosaic of resources, each with its own unique importance and contribution to the symphony of existence. These resources, which vary from the tangible wealth of natural components to the ethereal reservoirs of time, knowledge, and relationships, serve as the foundation for humanity's prosperity and advancement.

Nature's wealth is the most significant endowment, encompassing the oxygen we breathe, the water that sustains life, and the soil that supplies nutrition. Beautiful nature, rich in biodiversity, gives not only material riches but also mental and spiritual comfort. However, our continued exploitation jeopardizes the delicate balance, requiring us to embrace stewardship and establish sustainability for future generations. Time, an elusive yet vital asset, flows constantly, creating possibilities, moments, and experiences. Its scarcity instills urgency in our actions, encouraging us to cherish the present, learn from the past, and prepare for the future. Our lives are determined by how we manage and invest this finite resource, underscoring the importance of deliberate living and intentional endeavors. Knowledge evolves into an invaluable resource, transcending boundaries and opening up new perspectives. It enlightens, empowers, and encourages innovation. In an information-driven society, the ability to discern, synthesize, and apply knowledge is vital. Learning, when combined with practical application, strengthens individuals and civilizations, fostering growth and progress.

Relationships are a never-ending source of support, love, and companionship amid life's challenges. Attachments formed through familial bonds, friendships, and community ties bring comfort in times of adversity and magnify joy in times of triumph. Nurturing these connections, encouraging empathy, and embracing diversity enriches the human experience, giving us resilience and meaning.

The currency of health, which is often overlooked in the hustle and bustle of daily life, emerges as a valuable resource. Vitality, physical well-being, and mental stability serve as the foundation for productivity and contentment. Investing in self-care, emphasizing holistic wellness, and cultivating a health-conscious culture protects this valuable resource, allowing people to face life's challenges with vigor and resilience. Furthermore, imagination and passion, which are inherent in every person, inspire invention and drive growth. These sources of inspiration energize the human spirit, inspiring artists, businesses, and game-changing concepts. Embracing and developing these intrinsic abilities enables people to forge their paths, leaving an indelible mark on the world. The convergence of these resources creates life's symphony, presenting a plethora of opportunities and obligations. Our care as guardians of this treasure trove determines what legacy we leave behind. Cultivating a conscious knowledge of these resources, cherishing their essence, and properly using them benefits not only our particular paths but also the collective good of humanity. Let us walk softly in valuing the purity of life's resources, matching our objectives with the health of our planet and the flourishing of all sentient beings. Accept the richness of existence and appreciate its rewards, and you will become conduits for affluence, compassion, and long-term success.

Get moving: Exercise is a terrific method to enhance your energy levels. Even a brief walk might help you feel more alert and focused.

Stay hydrated: Dehydration can cause fatigue and sluggishness. Make sure you drink lots of water throughout the day to keep your body hydrated.

Eat a healthy diet: Eating a balanced diet might help you maintain your energy levels throughout the day. Make sure you eat enough fruits, veggies, and whole grains.

Get enough sleep: Lack of sleep can cause exhaustion and sluggishness. Make sure you get enough sleep every night so you can feel refreshed and energized.

 Get more sleep: Aim for at least 7 hours of sleep each night to boost energy and improve overall health.

 Reduce stress: Consider what is usually causing you to feel anxious or exhausted, and ask yourself if you can eliminate it from your life. If that is not possible or desired, what steps can you take to lessen your stress over that problem in the long run? Taking some time to relax, reading, or going for a stroll are all ways to boost your energy levels right now.

Stay hydrated. Dehydration can cause fatigue and sluggishness. Make sure you drink lots of water throughout the day to keep your body hydrated.

 Eat a healthy diet: Eating a balanced diet might help you maintain your energy levels throughout the day. Make sure you eat enough fruits, veggies, and whole grains.

Exercise: Exercise is an excellent way to increase your energy level. Even a brief walk can increase your alertness and focus.

Consuming too much alcohol might cause dehydration and weariness. Limit your alcohol intake to help you stay energized.

Take breaks. Taking a pause can be the most effective way to recharge your batteries. Spend a few minutes relaxing and clearing your mind. You'll return feeling energized and prepared to tackle your tasks.

Time, energy, attention, and money are examples of life's resources that you, as a person, can access. Making a list of your resources allows you to identify methods to make adjustments that will benefit you and get you where you want to go.

To give an example of a personal resource:

a. mentality: adaptability, resilience, growth mentality, self-awareness, self-confidence, and positive outlook.

b. Characteristics: sincerity, moral rectitude, compassion, kindness, tolerance, inventiveness, humor, and curiosity.

c. Competencies: teamwork, leadership, communication, critical thinking, problem-solving, time management, financial management, and teamwork.

d. Knowledge: instruction, practice, familiarity, competence, linguistic ability, cultural sensitivity, and digital literacy. Relationships: social media, networking organizations, family, friends, coworkers, mentors, and mentees.

f. Physical Resources: house, automobile, clothes, food, water, air, fitness, sleep, and health.

Increasing your resources can help you accomplish your objectives and create the life you've always wanted. The following

advice will assist you in enhancing your resources:

Time: It's critical to use time carefully because it's a limited resource. Set priorities for your work and get rid of time-consuming pursuits. Additionally, you can experiment with time-management strategies like the Pomodoro technique.

Energy: Vital resources include both mental and physical energy. Try to get adequate sleep, maintain a nutritious diet, and engage in regular exercise to boost your energy levels. Additionally, you can experiment with methods of relaxation like yoga, meditation, or deep breathing.

One of the most important human resources is attention. Remove distractions and concentrate on one task at a time to use it attentively. Additionally, you can experiment with mindfulness practices like journaling or meditation.

Money: Make a budget and follow it to increase your available funds. Another way to lower your costs is to buy fewer non-essential products. To help you increase your wealth over time, think about putting your money into a wide portfolio of investments.

Skills: Enroll in classes or workshops in subjects that pique your interest to develop your skills. You can regularly practice your abilities and acquire understanding from those around you. To meet people in your field, think about joining a networking or professional organization.

Knowledge: Read books, proceed to lectures, and enroll in courses in subjects you're interested in to increase your understanding. To extend your horizons, you can also look for new experiences and acquire knowledge from those in your immediate vicinity.

Relationships: Spend time with those who are most crucial to you if you want your relationships to be more proficient. Be willing to make concessions when required, and communicate honestly and openly. You might also join clubs or groups that interest you to meet new people.

- ## Harness the Power of Sluggish:

While it could seem counterintuitive, capital on sluggishness in a society that emphasizes efficiency and quick motion. But there's a secret power to seize the opportunity for stillness that can boost well-being, creativity, and productivity.
Harness the Power of Sluggish
The urge to remain constantly engaged in our hyperconnected culture can result in burnout and diminished productivity.

When deliberately pursued, lethargy facilitates periods of introspection. Cognitive rejuvenation It provides the chance to take a step back, assess, and gain a deeper comprehension of the tasks close at hand.

The idea of "slow living" has become more popular as individuals look for awareness and balance throughout their lives. It emphasizes the importance of living in the present, appreciating life, and taking time for personal use. This systematic approach can increase output by encouraging additional in-depth concentration and meticulousness when working on projects.

Furthermore, inertia might stimulate originality. When the mind is free to wander during idle moments, Many creative ideas come to mind. People can more easily access their creativity and generate imaginative ideas when they adopt a slower pace.

Significant benefits to mental health can also be attained by using indolence to practice mindfulness. Stress, worry, and a persistent sense of being overwhelmed are all lessened by it. Enhancing emotional well-being and developing self-awareness might result from pausing and continuing at a slower pace. Adopting a slow attitude undermines the value society places on being busy and emphasizes the need for relaxation and leisure. It promotes a change to a more sustainable and balanced way of living, where people are assessed on their capacity for self-care as well as their level of production.

Still, it's critical to find equilibrium. Accepting laziness does not imply shrugging off duties or going unproductive. To increase overall efficacy, deliberate inclusion of quiet times in one's schedule is crucial. It's significant to strike the correct balance between work and relaxation.

It can be rather than helpful to incorporate techniques like mindfulness, meditation, or just taking regular breaks to optimize the power of sleepiness. Making time for introspection and mindfulness regularly promotes brain renewal and improves decision-making. Being sluggish is frequently linked to being lazy or unmotivated. It could also indicate that your body and mind require relaxation and renewal.

Practice mindfulness: Being attentive helps you become more aware of your surroundings and slow down. To feel more focused and centered, try taking a few deep breaths or engaging in mindfulness meditation.

Remain hydrated: Being dehydrated might make you feel exhausted and lethargic. Throughout the day, make sure you're drinking lots of water to help keep your body and mind hydrated. A state of mind known as mindfulness is attained by concentrating one's attention on the here and now while kindly noticing and accepting one's emotions, ideas, and physical experiences. The following advice will assist you in cultivating mindfulness:

Locate a peaceful area: Look for a quiet spot where you may sit or lie down without disturbing anyone else.

Take a few deep breaths and concentrate on how your body feels as your breath enters and exits it. Refocus your attention on your breathing whenever your thoughts stray from it.

Observe your thoughts: As you bring your attention to your breathing, you can see ideas and emotions coming to mind. Keep an impartial eye on them and allow them to drift by like clouds in the sky. Regular practice is necessary since mindfulness is a skill. Try to dedicate a little period of time each day to mindfulness exercises.

Utilize meditation instruction: If you're new to the practice of mindfulness, guided meditations might be a beneficial tool. You can find free guided meditations on a lot of websites and apps. A mental health technique called mindfulness involves accepting the current moment and focusing attention on it. Among its many advantages are lower stress, decreased sadness, enhanced memory, and strengthened relationships. advantages of awareness:

Diminished depressive symptoms: A form of therapy known as mindfulness-based cognitive therapy (MBCT) combines mindfulness-based stress reduction (MBSR) and cognitive-behavioral therapy (CBT). Studies indicate that MBCT may be just as successful as antidepressant drugs in preventing the recurrence of depression symptoms, in addition to its ability to lessen them.

Enhanced emotional regulation: Mindfulness-based exercises can help improve one's capacity for emotional management. According to research, practicing mindfulness changes the parts of the brain that become active and inactive in response to inputs that elicit strong emotions.

Better memory: Being mindful can help increase working memory capacity, or the mind's capability to store and process information for brief intervals of time.

Reduced stress: By lessening the activity of the amygdala, a brain area implicated in the stress response, mindfulness can help reduce stress levels. Additionally, it may contribute to increased activity in the prefrontal cortex, a part of the brain related to emotional control and executive function.

Improved communication and empathy can result in healthier connections with others. Mindfulness can help with this.

• **Take Your Friction Off.**

The inability of one surface to roll or slide over another is known as friction. It only happens when two surfaces are in motion about one another. There are several strategies for lowering friction, such as:

Smooth surfaces: We could lessen interlocking if we made the sliding surfaces smoother. For example, a playground slide was polished to lower friction and smooth out the surface. Because there is less friction, kids can slide down a polished, frictionless slide with ease.

Lubrication: To lessen friction between surfaces, lubricants like oil or grease can be used. By forming a thin layer between the surfaces, they lessen friction and contact.

Streamlined body: In fluids like water or air, a streamlined body shape can help lower friction. For this reason, streamlined designs are used in the design of boats and airplanes.

Lowering the object's weight or pressure: Lowering an object's weight or pressure can aid in lowering friction. For instance, friction will be greater for heavier objects than for lighter ones.

Instead of using sliding friction, use rolling friction. Friction that rolls is less than friction that slides. Pushing a ball, for instance, is simpler than sliding it across the floor.

Instead of using dry friction, use fluid friction since it is less intense. For instance, walking on sand is more difficult than swimming in water. Eliminating friction means lowering the barriers that stand in the way of your success. For example, if you're trying to start an exercise regimen in the morning, sleeping in your training clothing will make getting prepared for a morning run or workout easier. Eliminating distractions and concentrating on one task at a time is another example. You can practice mindful attention use by doing this. To increase your attention span, you can also experiment with mindfulness exercises like journaling or meditation. Lastly, you can attempt to create a new habit a little bit simpler with these concepts that reduce friction.

Make a schedule: Creating a routine can assist you in spending less time and effort making decisions. You may focus on the task at hand and avoid having to make judgments about what to do next by establishing a routine.

Automate: You can save time and energy by automating tasks. To save time and energy, you may, for instance, hire a supermarket delivery service or set up automatic bill payments.

Organize your workspace: Maintaining an orderly workspace helps lower stress and boost output. Labels, storage containers, and other organizing supplies can help you maintain a clean, clutter-free workspace.

Use technology: You can reduce friction in a lot of aspects of your life by using technology. For instance, you can manage your spending using budgeting software or make meal planning easier with a meal planning app.

Assign tasks: Assigning tasks might help you make time and energy available for other pursuits. You can assign chores to friends, family, or coworkers, or you can hire an expert to assist you with household chores like cleaning or yard maintenance.

Reduce pointless commitments: You can free up time and energy for the things that are most important to you by saying "no" to pointless commitments. You can assess your obligations and remove those that don't fit your objectives or aren't necnecessary.

- ## **Acquire a lot of raw nutrients:**

Healthy eating often seems like a maze of options, but the core principle of eating well is still the same: prioritize unprocessed food. Whole, unadulterated meals are replete with these nutritional gems. They are vibrant fruits, vibrant vegetables, substantial entire grains, lean meats, and healthy fats.

Unprocessed nutrients have several benefits. First of all, they provide our bodies with a cellular feast of vitamins, minerals, and antioxidants. They strengthen our general health, boost immunity, and promote vigor. In contrast to their processed counterparts, these nutrients often come in a bundle with fiber, which aids in digestion and promotes feelings of fullness, which helps us avoid overindulging.

Let's go further to uncover the splendor of raw nutrition. Rich in color, fruits, and vegetables provide a range of health advantages. Phytochemicals, which are plant-based compounds with potent health impacts, are among them. Every pigment, such as lycopene in tomatoes and anthocyanins in blueberries, represents a certain health-promoting role.

Another important player in the field of unprocessed nutrition is whole grains.

Whole grains preserve their fiber, vitamins, and minerals, providing longer-lasting energy and supporting heart health, in contrast to refined grains that have had their outer layers removed.

Our bodies are made of proteins, and the best sources are unprocessed foods like lean meats, nuts, seeds, and legumes. These sources provide an abundance of essential amino acids required for hormone production, muscle repair, and general bodily functions.

Nutrient-dense, unprocessed fats from foods like avocados, almonds, and olive oil provide essential fatty acids needed for hormone balance, cognitive function, and the absorption of fat-soluble vitamins.

Adopting unprocessed nutrients is a way of life rather than just a diet choice. It means doing careful grocery shopping, selecting fresh produce, trying out different recipes, and progressively cutting back on highly processed foods. In addition, cooking with raw ingredients can be a delightful gastronomic experience. By experimenting with different cooking methods, home gardening, and farmer's markets, you can add variety and delight to your meals and turn eating healthfully into a fun ritual rather than a taxing chore.

However, convenience often lures us into processed, pre-packaged meals in our hectic world. These frequently have high concentrations of added sugar, salt, unhealthy fats, and other ingredients that eventually impair our health. But recognizing our alternatives and giving unprocessed options priority can be a game-changer when it comes to leading a healthier lifestyle.

To sum up, consuming an abundance of unprocessed nutrients is the first step toward vibrant health. It's about enjoying the pure, natural richness that our planet provides. It is a commitment to providing our bodies with nourishment from meals that uplift rather than deplete our well-being. So let's enjoy the benefits of a healthy, energetic existence by savoring the delicacy of unprocessed nutrition one delightful meal at a time.

fiber. Apples, bananas, oranges, spinach, kale, and broccoli are a few examples.

Nuts: Nuts are high in fiber, protein, and good fats. Almonds, walnuts, and pistachios are a few examples.

Meat: Iron, vitamin B12, and protein are all found in good amounts in meat. Beef and chicken are two examples.

Fish: Fish is high in protein, vitamins, and omega-3 fatty acids. The fish tuna and salmon are two examples.

Beans: Rich in vitamins, fiber, and protein, beans are a great food. Chickpeas and black beans are two examples.

Eggs: Rich in protein, vitamins, and minerals, eggs are a great food. They can be prepared in a variety of ways and are also adaptable.

Herbs and spices: Adding flavor to your food without gaining extra calories is possible with herbs and spices. Turmeric, oregano, and basil are a few examples. Increase Your Consumption of Meat: Even though meat is an excellent source of protein, it's crucial to eat it in moderation. Overindulging in meat consumption might result in health issues, including cancer and heart disease. But here are some pointers if you want to increase the amount of meat in your diet:

Opt for lean meats: Compared to red meats like beef and hog, lean meats like fish, poultry, and turkey have less fat and calories. They are a fantastic source of protein as well.

Veggie-Packed Omelets: Beatened eggs are cooked with a small amount of butter or oil to create a wonderful omelet. Add a variety of vegetables to it, such as tomatoes, bell peppers, mushrooms, bok choy, onions, and scallions. Omelets can be a great source of protein and nutrients. Oats don't have to be sweet—they can be savory! Try adding kale and mushrooms to your savory oatmeal. While mushrooms include protein, vitamin D, and vitamin B121, kale is a nutrient-rich food.

Make sure to include a variety of fruits, veggies, and healthy grains in your meals to maintain meal balance. By doing this, you can make sure that your body is receiving all the nutrients it needs.

Lettuce Wraps and Veggie Buns: Use lettuce leaves or specific vegetables in place of tortillas and bread. As buns use half-peppers, sweet potato slices, portobello mushroom caps, or eggplant.

Enjoy your favorite fillings in a calorie-efficient and delicious way with lettuce wraps.

Grilled Vegetable Kebabs: Arrange chopped tomatoes, bell peppers, onions, mushrooms, and zucchini on skewers, then sear them. These flavor-filled vegetarian kebabs are ideal for parties.

• Use Nutrients to Energize:

Maintaining adequate energy levels becomes a crucial goal in the fast-paced world of modern living when time passes quickly and demands never cease. During the process, it becomes clear how crucial a diet is to preserving health and vitality. The components of food and nutrition have an impact on our overall health, mental clarity, and energy levels. They serve as the cornerstone of all biological processes.

The macronutrients at the center of this intricate tango between nutrition and energy are lipids, proteins, and carbohydrates. To power cells and maintain biological functions, the body requires glucose, which is created from carbs through metabolic processes, as its primary fuel source. Proteins are made up of amino acids, which are building blocks that support the immune system, help repair tissue, and synthesize enzymes. Despite what the general public believes, fats are necessary for energy storage, hormone synthesis, and cellular integrity. The advantageous interactions between macronutrients and micronutrients, like vitamins and minerals, cannot be overstated. Vitamins function as catalysts in the pathways involved in energy synthesis, facilitating the release of energy from macronutrients. Minerals are required in smaller quantities, but they are crucial for the enzymatic reactions that are necessary for energy metabolism. For instance, iron is necessary for oxygen transmission, which has an overall impact on energy levels.

On the other hand, modern diets have undergone significant changes. People's fast-paced lifestyles are to blame for the surge in processed meals, which are heavy in sugar and unhealthy fats and lacking in nutrients. Due to this shift, there is now a paradoxical state of overconsumption and nutritional deficiencies, which can lead to a variety of health issues like fatigue, sluggishness, and weaker immune systems.

An effective diet must be carefully considered to provide energy. Eating a diet rich in whole foods—which are abundant in fruits, vegetables, lean proteins, healthy fats, and complex carbohydrates—restores the nutritional balance. A diverse range of nutrients is ensured, and a healthy internal environment is promoted by including a variety of vividly colored foods.

Beyond dietary considerations, another facet of the relationship between nutrition and energy is hydration. Water is commonly overlooked but is crucial for cellular processes. It facilitates the removal of toxins, the absorption of nutrients, and temperature regulation. Maintaining adequate hydration balances dietary intake and raises general energy levels.

Not to mention, it is crucial to recognize the significance of individual dietary needs. The degree of dietary specificity is highlighted by several factors, such as age, gender, level of exercise, and underlying medical conditions. Customizing eating patterns to satisfy these specific needs is necessary to optimize energy levels and promote overall well-being.

Mindful eating improves nutrient absorption when coupled with dietary modifications. Mindfulness has the potential to decrease overindulgence and foster a closer relationship with food by raising awareness of satiety cues. When one practices mindful eating rituals, such as observing textures, savoring flavors, and expressing gratitude, eating becomes a thoughtful experience.

Vitality is encapsulated in the symbiotic relationship between energy and nutrients. You can fully utilize the power of nutrients and embark on a transformative journey towards long-lasting energy, superb health, and a satisfying life with the support of personalized nutrition programs, mindful eating practices, and mindful dietary decisions.

Choose Complex Carbohydrates:
Whole grains, legumes, and starchy vegetables are good sources of complex carbohydrates. By releasing energy gradually, they avoid blood sugar troughs and surges.

Lean proteins such as chicken, fish, tofu, beans, and lentils are great sources of protein. Protein keeps you full, promotes muscle health, and aids in tissue regeneration.

Good Fats: Don't be afraid of fats! Pick olive oil, nuts, seeds, and avocado. Long-lasting energy and support for brain function are provided by healthy fats.

Hydrate: Fatigue can result from dehydration. Drink water throughout the day, and for variation, think about infusing your water with herbs or teas.

Foods High in Vitamins: Eat foods high in vitamins and minerals. Citrus fruits, bright fruits, and leafy greens are all great options.

Iron and B12, in particular, and iron are essential for the synthesis of energy. Add the lentils, eggs, spinach, and fortified cereals.

Snack Wisely: Choose nutrient-dense foods such as almonds, Greek yogurt, or hummus with vegetables.

Chapter Two

Goals and Objectives

Targets and aims define the direction we wish to move in, much as the compass points the way to success. These essential elements shape our aspirations by influencing our actions and efforts. They serve as the lighthouse guiding us toward our objectives, whether they be societal, professional, or personal.

Identifying Goals

Objectives that are specific and measurable and act as roadblocks on our journey are called goals. They provide a clear road map outlining the steps needed to accomplish our goals. Objectives, whether they are short- or long-term, are the pillars that support success. They provide us with a tangible standard to work for and measure our progress against, which contributes to a sense of direction and purpose.

A careful balance between aspiration and pragmatism is needed to achieve goals. Achievable objectives maintain motivation, promote further growth, and are reasonable. On the flip side, ambitious goals encourage us to push boundaries and get out of our comfort zones so we can reach our greatest potential.

The Value of Objectives

On the other hand, objectives address the broader, overarching purpose of our work. They elucidate the raison d'être or the fundamental driving force behind our actions. Our dreams, values, and ultimate ambitions are all included in our objectives, which are what drive us to work toward them.

By giving targets context and significance, objectives elevate our effort. They operate as a compass for us, guiding our decisions and actions in a manner that is consistent with our overarching goals and guiding principles. Goals provide the framework around which targets are constructed, logically directing our efforts.

The Relationship Between Goals and Objectives

Success requires that targets and aims have a mutually beneficial connection. While objectives are the specific steps needed to accomplish these goals, goals provide the general course. The alignment of these aspects is necessary to ensure that the pursuit of targets is harmoniously incorporated into the larger context of our aims.

Reaching a balance between short-term and long-term goals is essential. Short-term objectives represent baby steps taken toward long-term goals and act as stepping stones. They provide immediate focus and direction while keeping the bigger picture in mind. When we consistently accomplish these small goals, we gain momentum and confidence that advance us toward our ultimate goals.

Optimizing the Impact of Objectives and Goals

Setting goals and objectives takes thoughtful consideration, strategic planning, and a deep understanding of personal or corporate aspirations. Precisely defining these elements is essential, since it lays the foundation for an effective road map. Moreover, reaching our objectives requires flexibility. Circumstances shift, presenting both new opportunities and challenges. By establishing new objectives while staying loyal to your initial ones, you can be adaptable and resilient in the face of changing conditions.

a. Objectives:

Particular Objectives: Targets are exact, quantifiable goals we establish for ourselves. They lay out our goals for us.

Quantifiable: Objectives can be conveyed using numerical values, percentages, or other comparable metrics. Time-Bound: We have a specific amount of time that we want to finish things in.

b. Aims:

Broader Purpose: Our activities are motivated by our aims, which are broader goals or intentions.

c. Long-Term View: Aims are not constrained by time constraints, in contrast to objectives. They set the general course for us.

d. Holistic View: Objectives take into account values, vision, and influence in addition to the larger picture.

- **Deciding on a Target: A Thoughtful Journey.**

The act of establishing a goal signifies the start of a deliberate journey, acting as a compass to help navigate the complex routes of life. Aspirations, desires, and drives are woven throughout our lives, and targets are more than just places to be. Their importance goes beyond a simple destination; they become the embodiment of our goals, our aspirations, and our development.

1. The Origin of a Subject:
Goals emerge from a combination of willpower and vision. They frequently come from our needs, ideals, or passions. Whether it's reaching a personal objective, advancing a career milestone, or supporting a worthy cause, a target becomes the center of our aspirations and influences our choices and behaviors.

2. Accuracy in Objectives:
When defining a target, clarity is crucial. It's like putting coordinates on a map; the more precisely we can go to them, the

clearer they are. Focus is cultivated by precision, which directs our energies toward the goals we have in mind.

3. The adaptability dynamics:
Although they offer guidance, targets are not unchangeable. With all of life's turns and turns, flexibility is essential. Being adaptable in how we approach our goals makes space for development, education, and the acceptance of unanticipated chances that enhance our path.

4. Adaptability in the Face of Adversity:
Targets are not impervious to difficulties. There can be several barriers in the way of you reaching them. Resilience is fostered by viewing setbacks as learning opportunities rather than roadblocks. Resilience is what drives us to pursue our goals with unwavering determination, which makes our accomplishments all the more satisfying.

5. The Need for Satisfaction:

In the end, objectives are merely strands incorporated into the fabric of individual satisfaction. Reaching them results in a sense of fulfillment that goes beyond simply achieving the objective. Through this voyage and quest, we discover the core of our abilities and the full extent of our potential.

6. The Impact Ripples:
Objectives aren't only personal goals; they can have an impact on communities and beyond. Reaching personal goals frequently has positive ripple effects on society at large, serving as an example, inspirational, and motivating force.

7. Changing Objectives:
Our objectives change as we do. Things that were formerly important might become less important, be replaced by deeper goals, or be redirected as a result of shifting conditions. This evolution demonstrates development and the dynamic nature of human ambitions.

- ## **Target Hack: Strength and Cardio Exercise:**

The main goals of cardio exercises are to strengthen the body's cardiovascular system, improve endurance, and promote heart health. Exercises that increase heart rate include jogging, cycling, swimming, and aerobic workouts. This improves blood circulation and oxygen distribution throughout the body. These exercises help to increase lung capacity, decrease resting heart rate, and strengthen the heart muscle.

Cardiovascular training has benefits that go beyond the cardiovascular system. By burning fat and calories, it contributes to weight control by promoting weight loss or maintenance. Frequent heart exercises also improve mental health by lowering stress, anxiety, and depression and elevating mood by producing endorphins. To reduce plateaus and maintain motivation during cardiovascular exercise, variety is essential. Cross-training with a variety of activities, steady-state cardio, and high-intensity interval training (HIIT) may improve outcomes and reduce overuse problems. Strength Training: Conversely, strength training focuses on increasing bone density, muscular mass, and strength. It includes resistance training with machines, free weights, and body weight to push muscles and make them stronger and more adaptable. Exercises using resistance bands, weightlifting, and bodyweight exercises like squats and push-ups are a few examples. Strength training offers several advantages. Outside of training sessions, it helps with weight management and fat loss by increasing metabolism in addition to building muscle mass. Increased strength reduces the likelihood of injuries and age-related muscle loss while also improving posture, joint health, and general functionality in daily tasks. Furthermore, because strength training strengthens the skeletal system and promotes bone growth, it is important for maintaining bone health, especially in the prevention of osteoporosis.

Combining the Two: Although each form of exercise has its benefits, including strength and cardio training in a fitness regimen can improve overall health. This combination guarantees a comprehensive training program that raises overall physical fitness.

It is important to balance these two types of activities. Cardio and strength training can be done on different days, or they can be done together in the same session using circuit training or high-intensity interval training. This approach reduces training boredom while optimizing efficiency.

Furthermore, it's critical to incorporate enough relaxation and recuperation into the schedule. Strength training sessions give muscles time to repair and grow stronger, but cardiovascular exercises benefit from regularity without overdoing it, allowing the heart to adjust gradually. In conclusion, a comprehensive fitness regimen must include both strength and cardio training. Strength training addresses muscle development, metabolism, and bone strength, whereas cardiovascular exercise concentrates on heart health, endurance, and calorie burning. When combined properly, these two types of exercise have a positive effect that improves general health, well-being, and physical fitness. To fully benefit from a well-rounded fitness regimen, it is imperative to find a balanced timetable that incorporates both types of activities as well as appropriate rest and recovery.

Running combined with resistance training can help increase overall endurance, performance, and fitness. Research has indicated that integrating cycling with strength training can enhance muscular growth and strength beyond what can be achieved with strength training alone.

Resistance training and swimming together can help increase muscular strength and cardiovascular fitness. Resistance training combined with high-intensity interval training (HIIT) can help increase muscle strength and general fitness.

Enhancement of Cardiorespiratory Fitness: Recognize how aerobic exercise might improve your cardiorespiratory fitness.

Strength Gains and Health Benefits: Learn how strength training improves general health and muscle strength.

Create Your Routine: To improve your health, learn to design individualized cardiorespiratory and musculoskeletal workout regimens.

Of course

Time-Efficient Exercises: Marty and Stu offer exercises that may be performed almost anywhere, including at home, in a park, or even at your place of employment.

Keeping Strength and Cardio in Check: What is the ideal ratio of strength and cardio exercises? We answer this query as well as others.

Create Your Sessions: Discover how to create customized musculoskeletal and cardiorespiratory workout plans.

Martin Gibala As a pioneer of interval training, Marty demonstrates to us how to change up the intensity of our workouts to get in shape faster.

Stuart Phillips, a nutritional protein and muscle expert, highlights the benefits of using smaller weights.

Useful Advice

Anticipate enjoyable tests, engage in community involvement, and do homework to support your education. Regardless of how busy you are, make time for exercise.

- # Energy Level and Metabolism as the Hack Target:

Our metabolism and energy levels play a major role in our daily lives, affecting everything from our mood to our ability to function efficiently. The complex biochemical process of metabolism is how the body converts food and water into energy. This energy is necessary for many basic biological functions, including breathing, blood circulation, hormone regulation, and cell growth and repair.

The two primary metabolic processes are anabolism and catabolism. While catabolism breaks down molecules to release energy, anabolism uses energy to produce the molecules needed for growth and repair.

The basal metabolic rate, or BMR, is the quantity of energy required while at rest to maintain essential physiological functions. Many factors influence it, including body composition, age, gender, and heredity. For instance, whereas muscular bulk tends to boost BMR, age-related muscle loss may lower it.

The metabolism is greatly influenced by diet. During metabolism, various macronutrients, including proteins, lipids, and carbohydrates, release different amounts of energy. Carbohydrates are the body's primary energy source; they are converted into glucose for immediate use very quickly. On the other hand, lipids provide a more consistent source of energy, but proteins are required for tissue growth and repair.

Furthermore, metabolism depends on hormone regulation. Hormones like cortisol, adrenaline, thyroid hormones, insulin, and glucagon affect the synthesis and storage of energy. Thyroid hormones, for example, regulate the body's metabolic rate, whereas insulin regulates blood sugar levels.

Exercise has a major impact on energy levels and metabolism. Exercise increases energy expenditure, promotes the growth of muscular mass, and may even burn calories after a workout.

Numerous things affect metabolism and energy levels, such as stress, hydration, and sleep. Not only may sleep deprivation affect hormone balance, but it can also alter metabolism and energy levels. Extended periods of stress have been shown to raise cortisol levels, which may affect metabolism and lead to weight gain. Because nearly every chemical activity in the body involves water, metabolic processes must maintain proper hydration.

You need to live a balanced lifestyle to guarantee that your metabolism and energy levels are operating at optimal capacity. This entails obtaining adequate rest, controlling stress, eating a balanced diet in moderation, exercising frequently, and drinking lots of water. Modest, consistent lifestyle changes often have a cumulative effect on metabolic health. Numerous medical conditions might affect metabolism and energy levels. Inconsistencies that affect energy, weight, and overall health can be brought on by conditions like metabolic syndrome, diabetes, and hypothyroidism. Appropriate medical attention and lifestyle modifications can help promote the effective management of these illnesses.

1. Flexibility in Metabolism:

Our cells' ability to produce energy decreases with age. This deterioration affects our general vigor and hastens aging. Enhancing metabolic flexibility—the body's capacity to fluidly transition between burning fat and carbs for energy—is one effective anti-aging tip. We can slow down the aging process and sustain higher energy levels by improving this flexibility.

2. Methods of Biohacking: provides creative strategies for achieving goals with little work. Let's investigate a few methods:

a. Total Body Motion:

The potential benefits of whole-body vibration (WBV) to enhance metabolism and energy levels have drawn attention. Including WBV in your daily regimen can have a big impact. To improve your workouts, think about utilizing platforms or gadgets that offer controlled vibrations.

b. EMS, or electrical: muscle stimulation

Electrical impulses are used in EMS to stimulate muscles. It's a useful strategy for enhancing metabolic health and strength. EMS improves general fitness and energy levels by activating muscle fibers.

c. Humming and the Polyvagal Theory:

According to the polyvagal theory, humming can cause the vagus nerve to become activated, which would enhance the synthesis of nitric oxide. For both general health and energy metabolism, nitric oxide is essential.

d. Calm and Mental Well-Being:

Our general health is impacted by achieving mental clarity, emotional stability, and equanimity. For mental clarity and sustained energy levels, specific minerals and vitamins are necessary.

3. Not Harder, But Wiser:
Recall that maximizing health doesn't have to be difficult. We can do more with less effort and get longer-lasting outcomes by implementing biohacking concepts. Let's take advantage of our natural lethargy and make better decisions to improve our health.

• Hack Target: Brain and Neurological Fitness:

With billions of neurons governing every action, thought, and emotion, the human brain is a miracle. For general well-being, maintaining adequate brain health is essential. There are many aspects of neurological health, such as total brain fitness, emotional stability, and cognitive function.

1. Health of the Nerves:
The brain's amazing capacity to rearrange and adapt throughout life is known as neuroplasticity. Learning, memory formation, and injury recovery are all made possible by it.

2. Neurotransmitters: Molecular messengers that let neurons communicate with one another. Acetylcholine, serotonin, and dopamine are essential for memory, learning, and mood regulation.

3. Brain Structure: Specific functions are controlled by different areas of the brain. The hippocampus is essential for remembering, while the prefrontal cortex controls decision-making.

4. Neurological Disorders: Diseases that impair neurological health, such as epilepsy, Parkinson's, Alzheimer's, and others, frequently influence daily functioning and cognitive capacities.

1. Brain Fitness:

Mental Stimulation: The brain is stimulated by difficult tasks, puzzles, reading, and picking up new abilities. This process encourages neurogenesis and synaptic plasticity.

Physical Exercise: By increasing blood flow, stimulating neurogenesis, and lowering the risk of cognitive decline, regular physical activity improves brain health.

Healthy Diet: Diets high in vitamins, antioxidants, and omega-3 fatty acids promote cognitive performance and brain health.

Restorative Sleep: Restorative sleep is essential for brain health in general, emotional control, and memory consolidation. Good restorative sleep enhances mental function.

2. Programs for Brain Fitness:

Cognitive training: programs that use games and brain exercises to enhance attention, memory, and problem-solving abilities.

Mindfulness and meditation: techniques that improve mental health by lowering stress, sharpening focus, and fostering brain health.

Neurofeedback: methods that help people self-regulate how their brains operate, which can help with the management of disorders like anxiety and ADHD.

Brain-Computer Interfaces (BCIs): Developments that enable direct brain-to-external device contact hold promise for helping people with disabilities.

3. Improving Brain Health:

Maintain social engagement: social interaction boosts mental and emotional well-being.

Control stress: Prolonged stress can have a detrimental effect on brain function. Stress-reduction methods include deep breathing, yoga, and hobbies.

Lifelong Learning: Learning never stops, whether it comes from formal schooling or extracurricular interests. It keeps the mind sharp and involved. Minimize Toxins: Reducing exposure to substances such as drugs, alcohol, and too much caffeine promotes brain health.

1. Metabolic Adaptability for Mental Well-Being:

Our brain cells' ability to produce energy decreases with age, which affects our energy levels and mental abilities. Enhancing metabolic flexibility—the brain's capacity to fluidly transition between using multiple energy sources, such as glucose and ketones—is one potent Biohacking. We can enhance brain health and sustain higher energy levels by improving this flexibility.

2. Brain Communication via Wireless:
It was previously believed that nerve cells could only interact through physical connections, or "wired pathways." Nevertheless, new studies show that they can also communicate wirelessly by producing small electric fields. By enabling nearby nerve cells to detect one another's activity, these fields expand the network of neural connections. Observing these electromagnetic fields externally to the skull offers a unique perspective on nerve impulse transmission.

3. Brain Fitness Through Biohacking:
Methods
Now let's look at various biohacking methods to improve brain function:
Comprehensive Body Vibration (WBV)
WBV's ability to enhance metabolism and energy has drawn attention. It's

interesting to note that improving blood flow and promoting neuronal activity, might help improve brain health.

a. EMS, or electrical muscle stimulation:

Electrical impulses are used by EMS to activate muscles. It has benefits for metabolic health and brain function, in addition to physical strength.

b. Humming and the Polyvagal Theory:

According to the polyvagal theory, humming causes the vagus nerve to become activated, which increases the synthesis of nitric oxide. For both general health and energy metabolism, nitric oxide is essential.

c. Calm and Mental Well-Being:

Brain fitness is directly impacted by achieving emotional stability and mental equilibrium, or equanimity. A sufficient diet, which includes vital vitamins and minerals, promotes sustained energy levels and cognitive performance.

d: Establish Your Objective:

Establishing a specific objective gives your journey direction, just like when you draw a course on a map. Let's examine how to decide what your objective is:

1. Consider Your Wishes:

Give yourself some time to reflect. What is it that you want? Think about your goals, hobbies, and passions.

Consider the following: What would give my life meaning and fulfillment?

2. Establish measurability:

Calculate your objective. How are you going to know when you're done?

If your objective is to improve your fitness, for example, create a quantifiable goal like running five kilometers in under thirty minutes.

3. Establish a deadline:

Goals require a feeling of immediacy. If there's no deadline, they might
stay dreaming.
Choose the date that you wish to accomplish your goal. Will it be before the year ends? After five years?

4. See Your Success in Pictures:
Envision reaching the objective. What is the::sensation? How does one define success?
Visualization helps you stay motivated and concentrated.

5. Break It Down: Break your objective down into more achievable steps. These turn into your goals.
You grow closer to your ultimate goals with each target you reach.
Better Decisions for Brain Growth
Recall that maintaining brain fitness doesn't have to be difficult. We can do more with less effort and get longer-lasting outcomes by implementing biohacking concepts. Let's embrace our

natural curiosity and go deeper into the intriguing field of brain health.

• **Resilience and recovery are the hack targets:**

Recovery and resilience are aspects of human existence that support the ability to withstand, adjust, and eventually prosper in the face of hardships. They embody the innate human capacity to overcome obstacles, restore ambitions that have been dashed, and steel oneself against adversity.

Recognizing Recuperation

To put it simply, recovery is the process of getting back what was lost or adjusting to a new situation after a trauma, setback, or difficult situation. It covers a wide range of aspects, including mental, emotional, physical, and even spiritual. Its central concept is restoration, in which people work to bring themselves back into balance, find purpose amid chaos, and mend wounds, whether they are external or hidden deep within the soul.

The Complex Character of Healing

But the road to recovery is not a straight one. It's a maze of stages, each filled with its struggles and victories. It begins with acknowledgment, or admitting to one's hardship or misfortune. This recognition is the starting point for development; it creates self-awareness and ignites the initial spark of resilience.

The process then meanders through several phases, from reflection and introspection to proactive attempts at recovery. It requires perseverance in the face of adversity, patience, and fortitude. The trip ends in a changed condition where the wounds from the past are a reminder of the courage and will that are still present.

The Resilient Mindset

Conversely, resilience is the inherent ability to overcome hardship, adjust, and flourish despite it. It is the hope-filled light that shines through the darkest hours, fostering the idea that adversity is not an impassable barrier but rather a springboard for one's development.

Revealing the Components of Adaptability

Resilience is fundamentally influenced by a variety of elements, including psychological, social, environmental, and personal characteristics. It includes flexibility and the capacity to maneuver through strong seas. It feeds on optimism, fostering a cheerful attitude even in the most dire situations. Furthermore, a support network—whether it be friends, family, or the community—that offers consolation and fortitude during trying times promotes resilience.

The Relationship Between Resilience and Recovery

Although resilience and recovery are separate concepts, there is no denying their mutual influence. Resilience is frequently invoked in recovery as a catalyst, advancing people on their difficult path. At the same time, resilience serves as a pillar of support, enabling people to bravely and resolutely sail through the rough waters of rehabilitation.

Developing Recuperation and Fortitude

A diverse strategy is needed to cultivate these qualities. It demands introspection, the development of self-compassion, and an acceptance of vulnerability. It entails building a network of support, asking for advice, and lending a hand when required. It also necessitates the development of mindfulness techniques, adaptive coping strategies, and a growth mindset, which views setbacks as chances for improvement and learning. Although it can take some time and effort to develop resilience, it is a trait that can be acquired over time. The following advice can help you become resilient:

Discover your mission: Having a purpose in life may keep you motivated and concentrated when things get tough. Think about your objectives and values for a while, then consider how you may make your behaviors more consistent with these ideals.

Have faith in yourself. One of the key components of resilience is self-assurance. Try not to talk negatively about yourself; instead, concentrate on your accomplishments and strengths.

Create a social network: Being surrounded by a network of support can help you deal with stress and hardship.

Speak with your loved ones; think about joining a support group.

Accept change: Life is full of change, and being able to adjust to new circumstances can help you become more resilient. Strive to have an optimistic outlook on change and concentrate on the opportunities it brings.

Be upbeat: Being upbeat can help you keep a cheerful attitude even under trying circumstances. Try to see the bright side of things and seek out chances for personal development.

Nurture yourself: Maintaining your mental and physical well-being is crucial to building resilience. A nutritious diet, frequent exercise, and adequate sleep are all important.

Make time for enjoyable activities as well, including reading, listening to music, or spending time with close friends and family.

Develop your problem-solving abilities.
Being able to handle challenges well can
make you feel more in control and
confident. Develop your problem-solving
techniques by dissecting difficult issues
into smaller, more doable steps.
Set objectives: Having objectives will
keep you motivated and focused. Ensure
that your objectives are time-bound,
meaningful, quantifiable, achievable, and
specific (SMART).
Act: Taking initiative might give you a
greater sense of control over a
circumstance. Little actions can have a
significant impact.
Assist in developing your skills
gradually: Resilience-building is a
process that requires patience and work.
Resolve to gradually acquire these
abilities and practice self-compassion.

**1. The Healing Art of Injuries and
Wounds:** There are physical, emotional,
and spiritual scars left by life. Healing,

however, is an art. The goal is to turn wounds into tales of survival rather than erase them.

Resilience: Our ability to bounce back from harsh blows evolves, much like a tree. We don't break; we just bend. Every obstacle encountered becomes a springboard for improvement.

2. The Phoenix Within Rising from Ashes: After being consumed by fire, the fabled phoenix resurfaces. Adversity fires our inner phoenix. "You are more than your pain," it murmurs.

Resilience is the ability to dance through a fire and draw strength from the embers rather than try to escape it.

3. The Fragile Thread of Hope: Hope acts as a fragile thread amid broken dreams. It reassembles fragments to form a mosaic of opportunity.

Resilience: Hope is the unwavering conviction that dawn always comes after the darkest night. It is not naive optimism.

4. The Recovering Symphony

Notes of Courage: Healing is a team effort. It is a symphony, a product of our resolve, friends, and therapists working together.

Resilience: The song of resilience is added with every note played and every step ahead.

5. The Gentle Navigation Compass of Self-Compassion: Self-compassion serves as our compass. "You're human," it states. It's acceptable to error.

Resilience: Through self-compassion, we acquire the fortitude to get back up, pick ourselves up, and carry on.

Better Decisions for Brain Growth

Recall that maintaining brain fitness doesn't have to be difficult. We can do more with less effort and get longer-lasting outcomes by implementing biohacking concepts. Let's embrace our natural curiosity and go deeper into the intriguing field of brain health.

Chapter Three

Constant Improvement

In the wide world of human endeavor, there are no limits to the pursuit of improvement. This objective, sometimes referred to as "Infinite Enhancement," represents the unshakable dedication to constantly pushing past current boundaries and exploring new frontiers.

The Qualities of Advancement

The innate human desire for progress is embodied by infinite enhancement. It covers a broad spectrum of subjects, including science, technology, human development, and social transformation. It is the force that propels creativity and invention, pushing us beyond what we can do now.

Advancements in Technology

In the field of technology, the idea is simple to understand. Constant progress in artificial intelligence, biotechnology, space travel, and other scientific fields is a prime example of the never-ending quest for betterment. With every achievement, humanity surpasses earlier boundaries and creates a universe of hitherto unthinkable possibilities.

Human Ability

Not only is infinite improvement possible in the technological domain, Additionally, it also relates to the study of human potential. People and societies are constantly seeking innovative approaches to enhance their emotional intelligence, physical prowess, cognitive abilities, and general well-being. This innate drive for development is consistent with the objectives of mental toughness, education, and self-improvement. Consequences for Society and Ethics Conversely, the pursuit of infinite enlargement raises moral questions. It is imperative that we carefully negotiate the ethical terrain going forward. Fair access to inventions, the moral implications of new technology, and the social effects of rapid advancement are some of the issues brought up.

Managing Ambition and Accountability It becomes crucial to strike a balance between responsible innovation and aspirational advancement. To navigate the path of endless enhancement, one must cultivate a worldview that fosters innovation while considering its ethical, social, and environmental repercussions.

• **Power of the Spirit:**

Spiritual strength is an ethereal force that resides in the deepest corners of our being and helps us navigate life's storms. It's a mysterious yet profound quality that helps us grow as individuals and fortifies our resistance. At its core, spiritual strength is made up of several different traits that combine inner strength with purpose, faith, resiliency, and mindfulness.

Spiritual strength is fundamentally rooted in faith, which is an unwavering belief in something greater than ourselves. Whether grounded in philosophy, religion, or personal ideals, faith acts as a stabilizing force, providing comfort during trying times. It is the beacon of hope and fortitude in the face of adversity, shining brilliantly on the darkest paths.

Resilience, or the capacity to bend without breaking, is another essential component of spiritual power. It is the capacity to overcome challenges in life and come out stronger, taking lessons from them instead of giving up. Developing resilience means using inner resources to handle life's unforeseen currents and viewing change as a chance for advancement.

By fostering a closer relationship with both the self and the outside world, mindfulness, or the practice of being fully present in the moment, cultivates spiritual potency. It means developing self-awareness and inner peace by tuning into one's thoughts, feelings, and surroundings without passing judgment. Through mindfulness practices like meditation or introspection, people feed their spiritual core, bringing peace and clarity to the chaos of daily life.

Spiritual power is fueled by purpose, which functions as a beacon. A feeling of purpose guides actions and decisions toward a greater goal, giving life direction and meaning. It establishes a strong foundation for spiritual resilience by igniting passion, perseverance, and a sense of fulfillment.

Self-care and introspection are essential for spiritual development. Prayer, meditation, walks in the outdoors, and deeds of compassion are examples of soul-nourishing activities that replenish the spiritual reservoir inside. It involves recognizing the connection between the mental, spiritual, and physical facets of our existence and working toward a harmonious balance between them. Seeking spiritual power is not without challenges, though. Modern life is full of distractions that can block the path to spiritual fulfillment. Our spiritual viewpoint can be obscured by material aspirations, cultural expectations, and the never-ending whirlwind of daily living, drawing attention away from the true meaning of life.

Moreover, acquiring and preserving spiritual strength is a very personal journey. A person's spiritual boost may not come from the same source as another. It's a diverse landscape where a multitude of practices, beliefs, and experiences converge to generate unique routes toward spiritual fulfillment.

I. Resilience's Fundamentals:

Resilience is essentially the capacity to handle adversity and bounce back. It is the ability to change, develop, and flourish in the face of the most difficult obstacles in life. Strong coping mechanisms enable resilient individuals to gather resources, seek assistance when necessary, and devise solutions to handle challenging circumstances. They understand that they can persevere through difficult times and eventually overcome them. Resilient people typically feel that they have some influence over their destiny and possess a strong internal center of control. They take a logical approach to the problem and work to develop workable answers. Additionally, they are accepting of who they are and compassionate toward themselves, even in the face of adversity. Another indication of resilience is having a strong support system.

II. The Trial Anvil:

Imagine a forge used by an old blacksmith. The anvil, battered by innumerable hammer strikes, stands unwavering. The challenges of life, such as the weight of sadness, the scorching fires of loss, and the tempests that threaten to tear us apart, can give rise to spiritual strength.

III. Faith's Alchemical Process:

The furnace of faith forges spiritual strength. Not blind faith but knowledge, a confidence in the currents that run beneath the surface of our lives. It's the conviction that we all possess a cosmic compass that guides us toward our goals even in the face of obscurity.

IV. The Compassion Weaving:

Being strong is a team effort. It weaves together with compassion to form a resilient tapestry. We find our wings when we help others. Truly listening to one another's tales gives us comfort. Strength is the weave, and compassion is the warp.

V. The Stillness of Silence:

Silence fosters spiritual strength. We retreat into contemplation, prayer, or meditation to escape the cacophony of daily life. Here we are in contact with the eternal, taking our nourishment from the fountainhead of being. We gather pieces of eternity in silence.

VI. The Surrender Dance:

Ironically, giving up is where strength resides. Not failure, but submission to the universal current. We let go of our closed fists and let life's currents carry us. We give up control, believing the cosmos is working in our favor. We discover grace in surrender.

> **The Stars Inside:**
Resilience constellations shine within each of us. The stories of the fights, the tears, and the laughs are engraved in our bones. Spiritual strength is our entire galaxy, not just one particular star.
So, dear fellow seeker, bury this lesson deep in your heart: spiritual strength is a garden, not a stronghold. Treat it with care, kindness, and tenderness. Allow it to grow, blossom after blossom until you are a constant haven of light

- **Reaching The Next Level of Improvement:**

improvement. Upgrades are essential for our lives to go forward, much as technical advancements are designed to increase utility and performance.

It's often the case that moving forward requires embracing change, letting go of deeply held beliefs, and welcoming new perspectives. It's about pushing boundaries, seeking growth, and stepping outside of one's comfort zone. Upgrading is a deliberate choice to adapt, innovate, and increase our capacity.

The path to the next level is not without its challenges. It demands resilience, determination, and an unwavering commitment to personal development. Embracing the journey and all of the lessons learned, challenges surmounted, and victories won along the way is more significant than concentrating solely on reaching your goals.

It takes introspection to improve oneself. It's about realizing your strengths and weaknesses and using these insights as a platform for personal growth. It's about always growing as a person, picking up new skills, and honing ones that already exist.

The ability to adapt is also necessary for upgrading. Being adaptable is not only a decision; it is a necessity in the modern world that is changing so swiftly. The key traits that propel us forward are flexibility, openness to new ideas, and adaptability.

Making lasting relationships is more important for progress than only improving oneself. Our success is a result of collaborating with like-minded individuals, learning from other perspectives, and exchanging experiences. Together, we overcome obstacles and support one another.

People are often prevented from upgrading by anxiety. Our apprehensions about failure, the unknown, or moving outside our comfort zones can impede our progress. However, it's critical to view these fears as teaching moments rather than obstacles. Embracing discomfort can lead to unparalleled personal growth and education. Furthermore, upgrading happens on a societal and global scale in addition to an individual one. It means working to improve the lives of others, giving back to our communities, and trying to create a more equitable and welcoming environment for all.

I. Reaching the Boundary:

Imagine a doorway illuminated by the moon. It is positioned between the known and the unknown, between the remarkable and the commonplace. It takes guts to cross it—an unwavering conviction t6hat there is yet more to discover and develop.

II. The Growth Alchemy:

Upgrading is an alchemical dance rather than a straight-line rise. We compile our experiences, the highs and lows, and condense them into knowledge. We combine patience with boldness and inquiry with fortitude. We turn leaden times into golden epiphanies in this cosmic crucible.

III. How to Unlearn Things:
Like a snake shedding its skin, we shed layers to climb higher. We unlearn the scripts that constrain us—the worries uttered by society, the restrictions passed down from predecessors. We aim and paint with intention on the blank canvas of possibilities.

IV. The Aspiration to Mastery:
Mastering our selected domains is beckoned by upgrading. We immerse ourselves in everything, be it the science of compassion, the art of storytelling, or the dance of quantum particles. Among the stars and sages, we look for mentors,

soaking up their essence like sponges from heaven.

V. The Harmony of Echoes:

Pay close attention. We are the notes in the symphony, which is the cosmos humming. Harmonizing with cosmic vibrations is the essence of upgrading. We tune our emotions to empathy and our minds to curiosity. We are in tune with creation's pulsar beats.

VI. The Dilemma of Letting Go:

Surrender yields strength. We let go of attachments, such as antiquated beliefs and armor. Identity that no longer serves us is released. This holy release gives us wings. Weightless, we take off toward the next level.

>The Stars Inside:

Star constellations emerge within us. Every decision and insight adds a star. We are galaxies in motion, not immobile entities. Upgrading is the ongoing process of becoming—the stardust that weaves our essence—rather than a destination.

So, my fellow seeker, etch this fact into your soul: moving up to the next level is a cosmic dance rather than a sudden jump. Step bravely, but with caution. Let the moonlight lead the way, and may your footsteps echo across time and space.

• You Are You:

You are a complex mosaic made of the strands of your goals, feelings, and experiences that make you who you are. You are a singularly created symphony of ideas, desires, and dreams as a result of the interaction between nature and nurture. You are a complicated tapestry that begs to be studied, from the depths of your being to the subtleties of your expressions.

Your identity is the core of who you are;
it is the combination of your values,
beliefs, and ideals. It is the result of the
experiences gained, the bonds valued,
and the obstacles overcome. Your
identity shapes your choices and defines
your path, acting as a compass to help
you navigate the maze of life.

Your journey is a tale that unfolds in
chapters of growth and evolution because
it is so intimately intertwined with the
fabric of time. Each action, each failure,
and each victory adds to the story of
"you." It's a story adorned with happy,
sad, resilient, and self-discovery
moments that create a canvas full of
experiential colors.

Your reality is colored by emotions—the
kaleidoscopic hues of the human psyche.
Your soul's contours are shaped by
emotions, which can range from the
warmth of love to the sting of
disappointment, from the rush of

accomplishment to the anguish of loss. These experiences make you robust, compassionate, and utterly human. You are propelled onward by your aspirations, those shooting stars that illuminate the night sky of your goals. They murmur growth promises, inviting you to write your tale in the ink of tenacity and resolve, to embrace obstacles, and to reach beyond your comfort zone.

Your voice rises above the cacophonous chaos of the outside world, a monument to your uniqueness. Your ideas, beliefs, and thoughts are a mosaic of your reflections and outside influences that reverberate through existence, adding to the overall story of human consciousness. But you're also part of a bigger ensemble—the interwoven human web—within this symphony of individuality. Your actions, no matter how small, create ripples in this pool of shared existence, impacting the lives of people around you and making a lasting impression on society as a whole.

You must negotiate the conflict between authenticity and adaptation in your search for your identity. It takes constant work to strike a delicate balance between remaining loyal to who you are and changing with the times. This delicate equilibrium helps you define who you are while accepting the diversity around you. Fundamentally, "you" is an ongoing masterpiece, an exhibit in the human gallery that is always changing, reinventing, and growing into a new version of "you." Your essence is a complex story that adds to the rich tapestry of human existence. It is a blend of individuality and interconnectedness. Accept your individuality, treasure your path, and keep applying passionate, meaningful, and compassionate strokes to the canvas that is your life.

- ## Reviewing the Essence of Individualization and Duplication:

Both individualization and duplication are essential elements in many areas of life, including technology, personal growth, and other areas. These ideas each have their distinct qualities, but they also frequently cross in unexpected ways to provide new perspectives on creativity, customization, and duplication.

Personalization: Accepting Individuality, Individualization honors the distinctiveness that the idea that every human has unique qualities, experiences, and abilities that shape who they are. QIndividualization in technology drives customized user experiences that meet a range of needs and preferences. Individualization takes on a personal form when someone follows their passions and values their special abilities and viewpoints. It promotes acceptance of differences, inclusivity, and an appreciation of diversity's richness.

The Art of Replication by Duplication Contrarily, duplication focuses on reproduction, duplication, or recreating something that already exists. It includes the capacity to precisely and accurately duplicate components, procedures, or end products. In technology, duplication ensures consistency and scalability by allowing for the mass production of devices or the reproduction of data. Duplication is relevant to personal growth when it comes to following mentors' lead, copying successful tactics, or learning from excellent role models. It serves as the foundation for innovation, facilitating the exchange of ideas and methods among different fields.

The Crossroads: Where Duplication and Individualization Collide. Even though duplication and individualization seem to be at odds, they regularly come together to create synergies that spur advancement and creativity. This convergence is best illustrated by the personalization found in mass production when customized experiences are mass-produced to satisfy a wide range of preferences. Furthermore, technological developments enable the convergence of these ideas. For example, machine learning algorithms use user data to provide bespoke products or recommendations and then scale these customized experiences by applying duplication principles.When it comes to personal development, people frequently try to replicate success by modifying tried-and-true methods to suit their particular situation. Learning from mentors or role models entails copying effective practices while retaining one's uniqueness and sincerity. Ethical Issues and Difficulties The combination of duplication and individualization also raises ethical questions. In the world of technology, maintaining user privacy while creating customized experiences through the ethical use of individualized data becomes crucial. We need to regulate and carefully consider striking a balance between the advantages of personalization and the possible risks of exploitation. In addition, it might be difficult to walk the thin line between being honest and imitating success in personal development. Although copying effective tactics might be beneficial, it's important to maintain uniqueness and your development instead of just copying others.

1. The Echoes: Our subconscious hears repetition speak secrets. It etchings patterns and well-worn grooves into our neuronal circuits.We go over old routines, memories, and rituals again. Through sheer repetition, the commonplace takes on a sacred quality.But be careful—the echo chamber can magnify delusion as well as reality.

2. Alchemy: Wisdom is transformed from raw experience through repetition. It smoothes off sharp edges and highlights unnoticed details.We combine moments, extract significance, and condense essence, much like alchemists.But proceed with caution. Repetition too much hardens the soul.

3. The Mirage: Knownness is not always true. We take the well-traveled route for granted. Customized repetition obscures originality. It makes us oblivious to new directions and viewpoints.Explore the haven behind the illusion. Break out of the monotony's gravitational group

Conclusion:

The world is a wonderful place with a lot of difficulties and opportunities. We have to keep in mind that we are all in this together as we proceed. To build a better future for ourselves and the generations to come, we must cooperate. Kindness toward one another and readiness to assist those in need are essential. We also need to be open to growing as people and learning from our errors. By doing this, we can build a more equitable, prosperous, and peaceful world for everybody. With open minds and hearts, let's take on this task and collaborate to create a better.